Thou Art That

Thou Art That

Poems by Matthew Leavitt Brown

Cherry Grove Collections

Published by Cherry Grove Collections
P.O. Box 541106
Cincinnati, OH 45254-1106

ISBN: 978-1-62549-289-0

Poetry Editor: Kevin Walzer
Business Editor: Lori Jareo

Visit us on the web at www.cherry-grove.com

For Kathryn Grace and Richard Morrison,

for my family,

and, of course, for Ann.

You are the blue bird and the green one with scarlet eyes. You give birth to lightning and are the seasons and the seas.

– Shvetashvatara Upanishad 4. 4

Fear ye not therefore, ye are of more value than many sparrows.

– Matthew 10:31

And it is there,
      bouncing on the
            branch just outside
      the window on the tree
whose name you never

bothered to learn– Acer
      saccharum, for its sweetness.
           And you know, now, that it is
      you and that you are it
at the same time –

lifting slightly then
      settling, pure bright blue
           wind and weighting –
      forever, and ever
Amen.

Thou Art That

Fresh honey most mornings

I love you

Blue birds back outside our window, mating

I love you

Peony blossoms dripped with whitewash

I love you

Clean linens on clotheslines, blowing the backyard spring

I love you

Pink roses in a blue tinged vase
I love you

A hand carved tulip on the nightstand
I love you

Your chestnut curls for Sunday

I love you

The fine press of your gray skirt pleat
I love you

A white blouse untucked
I love

Late spring in mid-summer this year
I love you
Grandpa's rosary in the toolbox
I love you
Wind chimes pulling loose your name

I love

The soft shimmer of your eyes, winter mornings in the lake fog
I love you
Loose seed in the foyer
I love you
The feeder unfilled
I love you
The way I couldn't say goodbye

I love you

The first dishes of our own

I loveyou

The child we loved but never had

I loveyou

Little Emily waiting for her mama

Iloveyou

Your sweet breasts in the night air

Iloveyou

Your sweet breasts gone

Iloveyou

My ring's only mate, underground

Iloveyou

Small gray birds singing in the morning

Iloveyou

Iloveyou

You are gone

Iloveyou

Iloveyou

Forever forever

Iloveyou

Iloveyou

You are gone forever.

I love you. I love.

I loveyou.

You will be home when I get there.

You will be standing in the kitchen.

You will be wearing my grandmother's apron.

You will be laying dishes in the rack to dry.

You will have soap on your wrists.

You will be happy to see me.

Your hair will be tied behind your neck.

Your eyes will be clear in the evening light.

Your eyes will be lifted to mine.

Your eyes gone wet from corners.

Our song playing in the back room.

Our roses blooming the front yard.

My hands around your belly.

Your smile a lasting penance.

I will find you. Always.

Negley, Kathryn Grace – Age 33 of Randolph co., IL, died March 30, 2012 after a two-year battle with breast cancer. She was the daughter of Bill and Mary Greene. She is survived by her parents, her brother Thomas, sister Sarah (Lautner) and husband Morrison. After receiving her undergraduate degree in French from Illinois State, she taught English abroad in Paris, France, then returned to earn a Master's degree from St. Louis University. At the time of her illness, she was teaching in three county high schools. She enjoyed reading, cooking, gardening and spending time in the outdoors. She had a

lifelong passion for animals
and cared for several rescued
dogs and goats. Donations
can be made to the Southern
Illinois Humane Association.
A Funeral Mass will be held
at 11 a. m. on Tuesday, April 3,
at St. Francis Church.

She kissed him first on the side of the face where Cole Boys Creek runs under the old rock bridge that still stands, forgotten, next to and below the overpass that ends where the highway splits into eastern and western stretches along a strange bend in a river that runs from north to south. He can never remember how they had gotten there, or why they had chosen to sit, close for the first time, on a short set of stone-stacked stairs that once led to a house that had long since burned down. But he can, from time to time, remember the feeling of her closed lips pressed soft and briefly against his cheek. Her nose, which he had only found within himself the language with which to describe in economic terms as perfectly proportioned, and cute in the way a rabbit's is, flattened against the high, shaved arch of his cheekbone as she swept in and then out, like a child might kiss another child out of simple and unexpected impulse. And the light that came in through the arched stones of the old bridge from the streetlights that ran along the highway spread, under a forty-five degree angle of shadow, like a clean blanket of warm, washed towels that shone the trickling water the color of ripe sweet corn pulled new from the husk. It came through the small, dark opening in the way thin shafts of pale sunlight stream through heavy clouds in the evenings after late summer storms. It looked, he remembers having thought, like – if someone had taken a picture of them as she snuck her kiss, all that would have turned out would have been a hard patch of light, made of the darkness around it, holding within itself small glimmers of running water

that keep moving out, that keep moving out and away, that keep moving
out and away
and away and out
and away.

That keep moving and never come back.

Mornings —

12:30-Lie down

12:40-Turn on the lamp; Read whatever is close by

1:45- Turn off the light; Sleep

2:30- Wake up; Walk to the kitchen; Drink water; Drink bourbon;
       Drink water; Bourbon

3:00- Go back to bed; Read to sleep

5:45- Alarm

6:00- Get out of bed

6:00- Pace the house, waking up; Feed Whitey and let him out in the
       yard

6:25- Make tea; Eat cold cereal; Sit on the porch watching Whitey play

6:45- Shower; Shave; Dress

7:05- Leave for work

She is looking down, with her shoulder blades curled in the protective hunch a new mother might instinctively draw around the small curl of a new born. Behind her, groups of children are falling, mid-dive, into the concrete well of a backyard swimming pool as if the whole party had been choreographed for this moment. A small twirl of smoke is evaporating from a round charcoal grill into the limp sag of an American flag. Her face is bent too low to betray any emotion, but the child is looking up with the vacant eyes of someone either too young or too old to know who surrounds him. Her nearly bald head is covered with a spindle of blue and green cloth like you might expect to see in an African market or being worn by an old Russian woman. It was the last time they had been out together, in public. Later that night was the last time, too, he remembers every time he looks at the photograph that he keeps tucked in the middle of a well-worn copy of *Leaves of Grass* his grandfather left behind, that she had apologized for not being able to give him a family.

Because when he woke up, the color of her shirt was the same blue-algae color as the wall, so that when she sat up to blink twice and look at him as if she hadn't expected the world to feel like it did when she came back to it, the even plain of the room was interrupted by the dark shadows around her arms, the smooth auburn waves of her hair and bright blueness of the morning reflecting from her eyes. He felt as if he had, for the first time, been released into the fullness of his own body like a stone skipped across the moonlight of a large winter lake then sunk into darkness.

What's wrong, she had asked, still half asleep.

     – Nothing. I was just thinking about taking a picture.

She moved her head to one side and straightened her back. *A picture of what?*

     – Nothing. Nothing, Baby.

He looked towards the desk for a camera.

     – It's going to have to be a secret.

I can still see you, lying quiet
and small as the wind that lifts
cool through the grated slats
of the south bridge, just before
or after a rain in late summer.

Your skin, plum blossomed to
morning, swelled thick as honeysuckle
blooms the moonlight. The small,
sweet gap of your teeth. Your hair,
a growth of hayseed and lilac,

filled with tight nests of birdsong
and clover. Your bright smile
come easy. A body giving way.
The darkness, an unplucked string.
Your closed eyes, already given.

And if we have a boy, we'll name him Morrison, after you. And if it's a girl, we'll name her Emily, for my grandmother.

The sun came through the window and cut a diagonal line across the table from almost the middle to the corner on her side.

     – And why not Kathryn?

The sun came through the window.

Why what?

A diagonal line across the table.

     – Why not name a girl Kathryn?

Her face unlit, her arms, below the elbows, stretched in light.

Oh, I don't know. You have a Kathryn already.

The sun and the table moving. The sun and the table moving away.

And besides, I want you to have an Emily too.

The sun and the table. Moving.

I love that name.

She is turned, and smiling — eyes squinched against the cumulus-blocked sun, forehead tilted slightly. Irises, clear blue and solid as frozen river shoals but soft and slightly maternal in the way a young lover can be towards a young lover, looking slightly up towards the lens. And she is wearing a new dress; green, the color of alfalfa in late May before the first cutting, shaped wide in the neck and cinched tight along the waist in a fashion that made him think of his grandmother, snuck loose off the farm with a neighbor boy, or a peasant from a time he knew nothing about, but pitied.

Her hair, her long hair, the soft light color of buckeyes' inner ring, fallen in waves over her thin, bare shoulders with a few loose strands of curls falling out from the tuck behind her ear so that her face, though exposed, seemed withdrawn, as if she had been caught looking back, smiling, but absorbed in her own private thoughts — unstrung chords of lost chores and unfinished loves; vaulted things he cannot unlock. Stretched out in rows to her right, long braids of grape stalks blur into a shared mesh of dark green. To the left, a small red rose blossoms in an unfocused, burst. And she is twenty-three years old. And she is not his wife, alive though, as he ever knew her to be.

Emily unchained,
    Emily unbecoming –
        my baby, a tuck-kneed

peanut, unfolded from the soft
    pink tufts of her mother's belly
        swell. My greatest hope. I remember,

Kathryn, just back
    from the hospital, standing by
        the open moonlight in the window,

silent, while down the hall
    sheets tumbled, bleached un-bled,
        as the dryer buzzed with the sound

air should make, static-
    charged and promising
        an impossible spark,

while I sat on the corner
    of the stripped bed, fingering the air,
        wanting nothing at all, but maybe something

hard and mechanical. Something

    that needed fixing, something that I,

        through habit, could cure without thought.

Because today you have lain all day on the swing that hangs from hooks screwed into the turquoise painted slats of your uncle's summer cottage's screened in porch roof. And because you have been reading sheet music for piano from a few of Bach's preludes and the lyrics from a turn of the century Methodist hymnal as if they were linked chapters in a strange and codified novel. And because they are the only things in the house to read. And because there is nothing to do but sweat and laze where the bugs can't penetrate. And because wild columbine grows white and sunburst yellow in the shade of the yard that lines the driveway. And because the mountain breeze holds the weight of very old and hidden creek stones. And because you have paused, a few times, to hum out loud a tune that must have been blossoming in your head since morning, scaffolded in the chorus of other praises. And because I love you. And because when I do, I do forever.

Mornings –

2:00- Help Kathryn to the bathroom; Carry her to the stool; Lift her back to bed

2:30- Clean the mess in the hallway; Clean the mess in the bathroom

2:45- Don't go back to bed; Watch muted public television in the living room

6:30- Wake up on the couch; Check on Kathryn; Turn up the heat

7:00- Help Kathryn to the bathroom; Carry her to the stool; Lift her back to bed

7:15- Pills

8:00- Pills; Draw Kathryn's bath

8:20- Pills; Make breakfast; Dry Kathryn from the bath

8:45- Dump and wash the un-touched dishes; Pills; Put Kathryn back to bed

9:30- Dress; Check on Kathryn

9:55- Pills; Leave for work

And there you are, waiting,
the soft belly skin of your loose
body grounded across the bed,
a cursive unconstellation of stars
in my lonely night which ends,

always, where you are, but alone.
Your small starlight, a meteor of white
elements unburnt and light as the air
that lifts from room to room,
split by the passing of my body

towards yours, remembered as it
once was when I carried,
for your birthday morning,
a full bowl of strawberries,
picked fresh from our garden,

which grew as bright crimson

as the color you called "Christmas

Red" because they looked like the cloth,

hanging and lettered from the light-

poles under small colored bulbs

each December as we passed underhead

in cars at night, moving slow enough

to read the gold letters stenciled

under advent candles – *Ortum Dei*

Amen– driving down Main, fast as lost breath,

the blowing canvas flaps
lifted in the wind, streamed
against the sky, like one long
and open vein bleeding
the heavens, in a tight river, clean.

Because all that morning she was humming and singing the same tune under her breath, just loud enough for me to hear it across the house.

The way you wear, hum mmm…
The way you hmm, hmm mmm…

— And because I was hung-over after too much wine during dinner with friends the night before. And because I was on deadline and had to think straighter than I had allowed myself.

The way you, hmm, your hat…
You can't take that, hmm hmm…

— And because I walked into the kitchen and shouted at my sweet, my love, my Kathryn to shut-up and quit keeping with the same damn tune so I could get some work done. And because she stood straight up, surprised, dropped her face until her chin almost touched the small hollow of her neck, and cried without covering her face.

No, you can't take that away from me.

— And because I am still here, silent, and cannot let it go.

No, but really, do you think they'll like me?

She had asked this question without ceasing for the past four days.

     – Yes. I told you, they are going to love you.

She was sitting in the passenger seat of the robin egg blue, 1980 Toyota Camry that you sold a few months later for three hundred dollars. Your first car.

But how do you know that? You say it, but how do you know?

Her eyes, bright as the sky, and she looked directly at you in her twenty year old beauty.

     – I know, because I love you. I love you so they have to. No question.

You were driving on the river road then, past the barn where you had bucked hay as a teenager for a man whose name you don't remember, but who never paid you.

I don't think it works like that. I just don't know. I think they are going to hate me.

She brought her legs up and wrapped her arms around her shins, feet pointed towards you, leaning against the door.

What about your brother? He's going to hate me too.

Three horses were running in a field. You thought about the way the skin above the backs of her knees felt cool, even on hot days.

    — No, I told you that too. He is going to love you. Although, maybe not as much as he would if you were blond.
She faked a pout, stretched her right leg out and rested her bare foot in your lap.

I knew that's what you liked. I could go blond. I just never knew that's what you wanted. It might be fun.

You reached down and squeezed her foot, but didn't let go.

    — No, Kathryn is a brunette. Kathryn is a brunette, and what I want is Kathryn.

The first time they made love was in a single-wide one bedroom trailer deposited illegally on state wildlife reserve land by hunters to use in the cold afternoons of early December deer season. He had taken her camping, her first time, nearby, late on a cool Thursday in April. But when, in the middle of the night, a heavy rain had started up, rather than going home, he led her to the trailer, crawled in through a broken-locked window and let her in through the door. After spreading his unfurled sleeping bag over two pushed together aluminum cots, and covering it with the smaller one he had bought for her to use as a blanket, he built a fire in the scrap-iron box with a flue someone had welded to serve as a crude stove and heater. Once he stripped his clothes, save his underwear, and hung them up to dry near the flames, he slipped in behind her on the makeshift bed. That night they lay quietly, tracing the backs of their fingers across the embered glow of one another's tight young bodies, while he strung together whispered chains of every French word he knew in broken, nonsensical streams – *Me donne la baise. Me donne la Coeur. Je t'adore. Je te doit d'avoir. Je te doit* – while their bodies flowed and ebbed near togetherness. Until, in the earliest blue light of a spring morning storm, while fat goblets of rain patterned smooth waves across the aluminum roof in a way that made it seem as if they were all a part of one sound, happening as one, but unloosed from the falling forward link of time so that its singularity filled the room with a sweet, wet rhythm of impossible distance. And without realizing it, they found themselves pushing their bodies, hungry

and deep, one into the other, the dry canvassed

plain of his up-turned palms, the long arched

curl of her lifted back, the shallowing thrum

of her drawn breaths. The gray light

of rain darkened the black lines

that shadow every one thing from

another. And as she pulled her body

taut, and still, and he knew she was letting

go, he felt himself release and grow both deeper

into and away from the loneliness he had always known

and carried, and as it shuffled, he left it inside of her, where

he knew it would now always be. And he knew he was crying,

and that she was crying, small and quiet, and he wanted nothing more

than to apologize, and he did, again and over again, and he knew that no

matter how long he waited, their whole lives, together, there would never

be any language, for this, with which to say

I'm sorry.

She is half kneeling, just in front of the partially opened sun-yellowed garage door, with its dark and hidden collection of contents shining against the sun at odd angles, like a jack-o-lantern filled with random strips of tinfoil. And she is five, or maybe six, wearing a tiny white tee-shirt, red sweatpants that cut off just above the ankle and no shoes. Her hair, bobbed short, falls evenly down on either side of her head, shadowing the plumbed cheeks of her face below the cropped bangs as she looks down and reaches towards a small puppy, rolled over on its back. Her jaw is dropped and mouth spread wide in its light-red childhood fullness that has the same look as it would if she had just stumbled upon a cache of her favorite candy or a surprise visit by a real cartoon hero; a look that is greedy but forgivably so in its premature distance from self-awareness and therefore expected self-denial. And the scene is set at an odd angle, pulled just to the left, as if whoever captured it had done so without any kind of forethought. As if the entire moment had occurred and passed as unexpected and fleeting as the tucked lift of her very first puppy's black fluffed tail as it wagged for years beside her, and then, quietly, wagged no more.

You have been wrong,
    all these years, shoes
        piled in the doorway,
    dishes stacked above the sink,
yellow bones buried in the garden.

The sprinkler, waving
    the evening light, lifting
        children through clear wet
    beads like magic,
like the sharp sounds

they make when cool water
    touches their shoulders
        for the first time.
    Dragonflies landing
on reeds to mate in spring –

a wrinkled hand combing
    lake worn air, a spun line
        unwound above the face
    of waters that shakes the reeds
full of deep lonesome wild –

the red prism of their eyes,

    flashing the twilight to glaze,

        the hollow thrum of wings,

    calling you back,

leaving your body.

Shhhhhh she hushed, more a breath than something said. *Shhhhhhhh*.

— No, that's it. I know it now. That's why I want to marry you.

Shhhhhh. Her breath was even with her hushing, as if she were, instead of trying to quiet him, simply breathing out through her lips, which were swollen from pressing hard against his, covering her teeth in a different, but somehow closer, way.

— Oh yeah, I mean it. We'll get married, and then someday, after I die, and then you die, we'll have to be buried next to each other.

Shhhhhh.

— And you won't get a choice. You'll have to stay there, and we'll lie like this forever.

He moved up and lay down on his back next to her and stretched his bare legs and arms straight down, above the sheets, as if he were a corpse, as close to her as possible.

Shhhhhh. She rolled over towards him on her right side and rearranged the sheet tucked under her arm so that, with or without noticing it, part of her left nipple's darkness rose above the cuffed cotton edge where he could see it without moving much.

Don't talk about that. You don't know me well enough to marry me. She brushed over the features of his face with the tips of her fingers without opening her eyes. *And besides, I don't think you're ever going to die.*

He relaxed his body.

      — Why do you say that?

I don't know. I just can't imagine that happening, or you getting old. She reached up and pulled his face to the side towards hers. *Shhhhhhh. Listen.*

He lay still then reached up.

      — And I'll see if they can cut holes in the sides of the coffins so we can hold hands. So our bones can hold hands.

He tied her fingers between his.

      — Forever.

It is in black and white, late summer with the leaves on the trees heavy yet brittle looking in the background. And we are standing next to each other, your left arm wrapped around my waist, your right hand disappeared inside the blazer I am wearing that I took from my grandfather's closet when he died and left on a subway car somewhere under Manhattan for a homeless woman you thought looked cold in her stained and threadbare sleeping bag.

Your hair, blown free of the clip you had placed it in that morning when we woke up in an old elementary school converted into a bed and breakfast, curling around your smile like a loose wreath of dark silk ribbons. My face, clean shaven and bright, barely old enough to buy a drink. And we are standing next to a pick-up truck and a low wire fence on the ferry that runs two cars or one piece of heavy farm equipment at a time back and forth across the river just north of here.

The water, the color of wet and frozen ash, flush with broken eddies. The sky, an unrolled sheet of blank newspaper. The half-shadow of the ferry boat captain, a boy years younger than even we were, his arms folded around where his face would be, where he held the camera, looking like he was lifting his head above his body, like his wrists grew directly into his temples. And we were watching, caught in a moment of disembodied joy and amazement, carried back toward the dark swallow of the tree lined shore, away from the unseen mirror of another, pushing water into tight little waves that ripple out, farther down with the current than up against it.

Is it ok?

The oil from the unseasoned tomato paste, poured from a can on top of mostly drained spaghetti noodles, pooled in dollops in the left-over water standing along the rim of the bowl. Black flakes of carbon from the butter saturated and over-cooked bread were sprinkled around the table surrounding the placemats.

— No, it's fine. I just don't have much of an appetite.

He took a long drink from the juice glass, almost set it down, then drank the rest in one large swallow. The wine had come from a box and tasted like sugared vinegar after having sat out for over an hour before dinner.

— I'm pretty sedentary, you know, at the office these days.

The television, left on in the back room, announced a new batch of rain showers.

It's alright.

The skin on her face was tight the way a kitten's must be under its fur.

It will get better.

Kathryn drifted,
    Kathryn still alive —
        crouched on the toilet

loosened as a black wave,
    tideless. A small fissure
        in the shingles sending

sunlight through
    the attic, filling bare
        corners with damp rot.

Kathryn undaunting,
    Kathryn grown hairless —
        bare chest gone, sunken,

sweet skin one
    long fine wrinkle.
        And my hands,

pulling the earth up
    through the roots
        in a corner of our yard

I told her I would fill

    with perennials, the subtle prayers

        of nature, for her to tend next year.

My heart, husked

    as an untrue secret,

        and she will not make it.

Over the intercom, a man's voice announces a coming departure and two gate changes in English then repeats the same message, you assume, in French. Crowds of people rush by, silent and cross, fumbling with over-sized and overstuffed luggage.

It's only a year. And you'll come for two weeks over Christmas, so it's more like eleven and a half months. It really won't feel that long, I promise.

She is wearing a blouse that is the color of early morning light after a first frost. You, for reasons you still cannot name, are dressed up in a crisp white shirt with a suit jacket and a tie.

Please don't be mad at me. You know I have to do this. I'll never get into grad school if I haven't lived there. We talked about this. Please don't be mad.

But you can't trust your voice to respond. Tears stream down your face in thin lines that outline the corners of your mouth. The security line lurches forward. In a moment, you will have to duck out, under the black ribbons that separate the three groups.

I'm sorry. I'm sorry. You know I don't want to leave you. I never want to leave you. I'll never do this again.

The line moves forward.

You have to tell me it's ok. You have to tell me it's ok for me to go without you. Please. You have to tell me.

It is time. You say nothing.

The first time she kissed him

      the wind folded

           back the trees. The thin yellow

                light on the creek

                    braided itself into

                        the strained tune

                            bees make inside a hive,

                      northern ice split in half.

                Her breasts,

            swelled

        in the darkness. His mouth,

    a blank syllable

of loss.

Unrepentant.

I'm sorry, her face crinkled like soft peach tinfoil, like it was made of magnolia blossoms. *I'm sorry, I didn't know.* She knotted her fingers together and started to cry without covering her face, something she did often that he had never seen anyone do before — something that terrified him about her.

I'm sorry. I never... And he can remember this, what she said and how she looked, her hair pulled back into a tight bun with a few strands shaken loose, floating back and forth across her face, with her giant eyes blinking blue in the bedside lamp's quiet burn. Their bedroom, he believes, was arranged just as it is now, without her, and she was wearing a slightly tinged white undershirt they had bought in bulk and shared, a little too big for her, a little too small for him.

I'm sorry. She was crying and curled up next to him, wrapping her arms around his chest. And he can't remember what it was all about; why she was apologizing or what he had said in response. She wrapped her arms around him and squeezed her fingers together as if she had to hold him down, as if she was afraid that he might have gotten up and stormed out if she had not stopped him. And he keeps it with him, her questionably prompted tears and his slavish silence, and he carries it with him, wishing more than anything not to understand, but simply to forgive, and be forgiven.

She is lying on a bed, in a hospital room, covered with a thick mound of white blankets. Outside the large window, which spreads from her hips to the edge of the frame, a red glow blooms gently around the dark outline of a city's tall buildings, although he doesn't know where, exactly, they were. And her right arm is stretched along her frail and wasted body with IVs stuck in the back of her hand, which is turned to the side with the fingers curled in and thumb stuck upward. And she is almost as pale as the antique eggshell paint on the walls, reflected from the flash, as she smiles a small, tight-lipped curl of the mouth.

And she is wearing a turban that he made by wrapping a towel around his leg and rolling it down toward his knee because he knew, without her having to say it, that her bare head was cold.

Where did you learn to do that? She had asked while he tucked in the edges and reached over to place it on her head.

     – I don't know. Swimming lessons I think.

Did you learn to swim in the Red Sea? She had smiled then and sunken a little under the weight of the towel.

– No. Public lessons. But you can be my sultana so long as you keep that turban on.

Hmmm. She smiled and reached her arms out toward him without opening her eyes. *I think I'd rather be your concubine, if that's alright.*

He lifted the blankets and stretched out next to her on the bed.

– I'm sure that can be arranged.

Mornings—

2:00- Wake up in the hospital lounger, body ached, next to her bed; Re
       member dreamlessness
2:10- Walk to the nurses' central floor station for coffee; Listen to a few
       jokes; Pretend to listen; Pretend to laugh
3:30- Read the Gideon's edition left in the drawer below the latex gloves;
       Finger the peeling American flag sticker curling from the inside
       back flap
6:25- Wake up sweating but grounded, the sun in the room, Kathryn still
       asleep
7:00- Talk to the nurse on rounds; Watch her change the glucose and
       bedpan; Listen as the room grows light
8:00- Walk to the cafeteria for coffee and toast; Pace the gift shop; Con
       sider buying flowers; Steal a paper from the waiting room
9:45- Wait for her to wake up long enough to talk; Carry the paper back
       to the lobby, unread; Call the office to take another day off work
10:00- Wait for word from Kathryn

And she is there, wearing a dark blue batter's helmet, scuffed dull with use, hands choked a good three inches up the bat, splay-legged and facing a pitcher whose mess of blonde curls tufts out beneath the sides of her hat. Her rail-thin, thirteen-year-old frame is balanced under the weight of her arms, lifted as she waits for a rounded pitch. The dirt, stained on her knees, spreads up her thighs and brakes in crumbles above her ankles. Her teeth are set and clinched in the way they always were when she was set before a task she knew she could accomplish but had not yet fully set herself upon. And there is a chain link fence, unfocusing the frame in rows of ties in the foreground. Behind her, a row of bleachers sits empty and washed out in the afternoon sun. A thin stream of smoke blurs the bottom right corner where another father must have waited, smoking in the mid-summer haze. And it is faded, the way a picture that has hung for years on a refrigerator door should always be.

Hello, I'm Kathryn. I'll be your server tonight.

The wood-grain panel walls round the bar. Orange vinyl booths tacked to the east studs. Two gray men drink coffee from porcelain cups in the rear.

Hello, I'm Kathryn, I'll be your server tonight.

Against the shadow tinted sidewalk, neon letters spell out, backward, PUOS TOH, backed by a black box that buzzes its way to the outlet through a two pronged chord.

Hello, I'm Kathryn, I will be serving you tonight.

Her chestnut hair, pulled to a clip behind her round ears.

Hello, I'm Kathryn, I will serve you.

Her white collar, washed to a fray around her slender neck. Her bright eyes, large and blue as December storms the morning.

Hello, I'm Kathryn. I will be with you.

Cars back up the four-way stop outside. A single, blinking bulb. Old folks heading home, again.

Hello, I am Kathryn. I will be here in the morning. I will soak the salted earth in spring.

The street lights blink on. The hemlock groves bough to silence while forests sleep. The moon skinnies the tide, too low, toward peaceful.

I am Kathryn. I will be a pocket the winds keep to gather strength. I will be the honey that nectars bees to pollen. The pine needles that carpet the neighbor's drive will spell my promise to fall. My breath will matter the great darkness.

A row of empty chairs. A tip jar by the register, too empty. A deep thaw below the arctic.

An empty storefront. A business, no longer there. The first time I saw her, across the room.

I will give you reasons to have been born.

A loaf of bread, half gone, on the counter.

Peanut butter and three cans of condensed soup in the cupboard.

Mustard and spoiled apples in the fridge.

Empty bottles in a box on the drive.

One plate and a bowl in the sink.

The table covered in loose papers and boxes, untouched.

When you eat, you will do it standing up.

Negley, Kathryn

Grace – Age 33 of
Randolph co., IL, died
March 30, 2012 after a two
year battle with breast
cancer. She was the
daughter of Bill and Mary
Greene. She was the first
warm wind in April.
She was the sun cresting
the east field hill, the blue
light below the glacier.
She is survived by her brothers
and her sisters. She is survived
by the fir forests of the north,
by the light broken through
church windows, by the two young
appaloosas down the lane
who bow and paw the loose
earth each time you pass,
slowly. She is survived by
her husband. She is left
in the bag of green apples

she kept on the back floorboard
of her car so she could pause
and say hello when she saw
them by the roadside.
The one she called Dot after
the gold flecks running down
its legs. The one she called
Buddy by instinct. She is
the thing you miss when
you are not alone.

Just this morning, pulling weeds in the backyard flower garden, one and then two more baby bunnies, too young for sight, inched out from beneath the tight dark bulb of overgrown iris stalks, all three crawling into my upturned right palm and shivering. My hand, which must have sounded like their mother's teeth chewing through shoots of grass and broadleaves as I pulled stray weeds from the chipped cedar mulch, unexpectedly filled with life beyond recognition. And without thinking I called your name once, almost without making a sound, then again, louder, with my head turned back over my shoulder toward the empty house.

The first time they made love he felt his name stitched inside hers, each syllable patted small and unassuming as the unlettered chain of his breath-puffed clouds of air and water condensed islands of refracted light across the windows. Each short pulse, every hard pull of two bodies becoming – the blood rim of a dogwood bloom in spring, the dropped heart of March violets, a twin channeled dust trail that at one point, a long time ago, forded the creek on its way home.

And you are not there, spread
across the bed, waiting
in the moonlight for me to come.
And you are not there.
You are not there. You are not

there. You are nowhere. And I think
of your body, now, a year later –
its long browning, the lonely hum
of its sinking. And of whoever it was,
a man I'm guessing, though like to think not,

who first took you, after you passed,
and stripped you bare and washed
each of my favorite lost inches,
and held what was left of your naked weight,
and the cold steel table upon which you lay,

unfeeling and unfilled and dressed, a soft yellow
        dress your grandmother had made you
when you were a little girl
        that once again fit your starved and eaten body,
                that you said reminded you of the way the backs

                of sunflower petals looked, in your neighbor's field
        from a distance. And the way you turned to me, once,
just after the first diagnosis, and asked
        me to promise to never let you be buried
                in a wig. Then later, only a few days before you died,

you told me you didn't really care about the wig,
but wanted to wear your grandmother's yellow dress,
and I promised, but couldn't talk about it with you, not yet.
And you are not there. And you are not there, and you are
nowhere, and I am left with the hard fullness that
forever leaves.

She is standing thin, midstride and turning back toward him just off the Pont de l'Archevêché. Her eyes blinking in the snow, the black collar of her coat pulled up over her neck and ears like a sharp angled and incomplete hood. Beyond her, the gray faces of the Left Bank's cafés, boutiques and apartments open like a thin chasm of space that leads either towards or away from heaven under the navy black sky that holds clouds full of winter storms and foreign phrases that can be said only, or so it seems from her gaze in the photograph, in a very old city. Down the street from where she will exit the bridge is the fifth-floor apartment near the Fountain Saint Michel in which she rented a room for the year after they graduated college. A place to which he came to visit for Christmas, where he could watch, each morning, short men unfurl the yellow awnings of bookshops and boulangeries lining the cobbled street below her balcony, feral cats that live on the rooftops and never touch the ground chasing pigeons along the gutters, the man who makes a living eating cigarettes and nails for the livid fascination of tourists claiming his space for later. And she is in the process of saying something, her small ungloved hand reaching back to catch him, as if she was worried he would not be able to see what she saw if he was not close enough to her. And she is happy, but distant in a way he knows he'll never understand.

Because on the way out of town this morning she saw a possum writhing on its back by the side of the road, mouth open in what looked like an upside down half grin half gasp, splay-toed feet combing thin air for the ground, its bald tail wound tight around the round belly. Across the street a blank faced boy wearing oversized and open camouflage overalls watched the car approach then pass without moving his head.

Oh my God, her face pulled into sharp lines from within. *Is it really hurting?*

     — No. I don't think it was actually hit. It was probably just scared of something, that boy maybe. They release a pheromone, you know. "Playing possum." Remember?

She looked at her hands and turned them once backward then forward in the air in between her face and the dashboard for no apparent reason. Her expression unchanged. He couldn't tell if she was listening.

     — It takes them awhile to wake up and walk straight afterward.

And because that night, on the way back home, a wide arch of blood in the gravel by the roadside, no possum and Kathryn asleep, he thought, in the passenger seat.

You see. That's why I don't like to leave the house. Her eyes still closed. *You can't go anywhere.*

The headlights on the striped lines reflected, street signs shining in the distance, the terrifying and honest way, he could never name, wild animals fight to die alone.

She drinks moonlight back to glowing.

From Heaven, stars pour honey in her cup

and lift the oceans to high tide. Her bones

are soft and filled with birdsong and feather

duff. Her eyes munch the softest edges of snow

from among the firs. Hibiscus blooms honeysuckle

the way she says my name in morning.

Her plate is covered with wild heather

and paint from the southern desert

skyline, rimmed with tangerine and blackberry.

Water moves through her bowl and seasons the

sea to fullness. Her lips cover the

city streets

in daylight and carry me safe through midnight.

Such tenderness. Her taste is made of words

you couldn't say, but always knew. My Kathryn.

I love you.

She is grainy, flecked with the pocked air newsprint leaves when it is cheaply printed and mass produced. The plaid, western style shirt she is wearing was an impulse purchase from a roadside tourist shop outside Moscow, Idaho, where children can buy nuggets of fools gold, plastic, old-west sheriff badges and faux leather moccasins. He had picked it because it was the only picture he had in which she is looking directly at the camera while smiling. Beside her, which had been cropped out for the obituary, was a mule with its head turned away in a posture of well-practiced, non-violent protest. Its ears were lifted like those of a cartoon rabbit and were splayed in a posture that indicated a wildness that is only known by those who are well taken care of. In his copy of the picture, her hair shines with vibrant, earthy glow of a young woman who is healthy, content and fully at home in her own body. In print, the washed-out smallness of her face is uncolored in the mute drab of blank paper. Beside her eyes are thin ribbons of inked lines. A sign, he believes, that her smile is real.

You will be home when I get there.

When I get there, standing in the kitchen.

Standing in the kitchen, wearing my grandmother's apron.

Wearing my grandmother's apron, laying dishes in the
rack to dry.

Laying dishes in the rack, soap up your wrists.

soap on your wrists, happy to see me.

Your face blushed with happiness, your hair will be tied
behind your neck.

Hair tied back, your eyes will be clear in the evening light.

Your tied hair, your clear eyes lifted up to mine.

Your eyes, clear and wide cold blue, gone wet from the
corners.

Your soft smell in the kitchen, our song playing in the back room.

A soft whistle in your breath, roses blooming the front yard.

The garden gone petal pink, my hands around your belly.

Holding true your poise, your smile a lasting promise.

When you come back, I will be waiting. Amen.

Mornings—

5:45- Still asleep, together, legs hooked as links in a fleshed chain, a soft braid of quilted shadow and fresh smooth light
6:00- Wake up before the alarm; Reconnect, her arms wrapped around his shoulders like the locked clasp of a hooded shroud
6:20- Make love, lazy at first, then finishing strong; Open the blinds; Lie together in the early spring bloom, happy
8:00- Shower; Dress; Coffee
8:30- Kiss; Leave for work; Plan dinner on the phone during the drive

I think that's it.

She lays the brush on the edge of the roller tray so that only the tips of the bristles sink into the paint and pushes the hair out of her eyes with the back of her wrist, still streaking her forehead with a thin blue stripe she has tried all night to avoid.

"You think it's what?" my brother asks, trying to scoop the particles of ash that have fallen from his cigarette into his tray with a putty knife. He is tired and sounds disinterested after painting all night and helping load our things into a rented truck and moving all day.

It's the same blue that when I was a little girl I thought ocean water was. See? She picks up a color sample card and reaches it out toward us, pointing up toward the signature color title 'Pacific Swell'. *I used to think that if you went to the ocean and filled up a glass the water would be blue, just like this.* After looking around the piled folds of plastic and canvas drop clothes she finds her beer and takes a long drink, rolling the dried latex between her thumb and index finger. *I thought that the water itself was blue like this, you know what I mean, that you could take it with you in a glass. I used to ask my dad about it, but he said the water itself isn't blue, it just looks that way when there's a lot of it together.* She picks up the brush and paints clean lines around the window trim without tape for a long time without saying anything more.

I couldn't understand, as a kid, you know, I was just a little girl, how this could work. I used to ask him where the blue comes from if the water isn't blue. 'I don't know,' he said, 'it's just kind of there. It has its own blue, it comes from inside.'

She steps back to look at the window she has just trimmed to check for any mistakes she knows she did not make.

My wife, painting the walls in our new home. My brother, barely listening, prying the lid off a new can with an antique letter opener.

I never could understand what he meant by that.

And you believe, still, as you walk,

that sunlight, washing your skin warm

to afternoon, is the way she reaches out,

even though her body is curdled as spoiled

milk beneath the ground. You stop on the rocks

laid along the dammed lake shore by the Army

Corps of Engineers and feel the heat blister your

face. A blue heron takes notice and lifts the shoals

across the water. Her pretty bones petrify

to amber within the earth, while a mottled,

brown mallard gathers her ducklings into a pod

before you. They paddle away in a thin line,

leaving a dark blue trace in their wake.

Above the water, each small ripple separates

itself into singularity, the way you have

always known the world to be, held

together only by one clear light.

Because early that morning, just as the sun was beginning to stream through their parlor window, she found him asleep on the couch, caught in a swirl of yellow and blue post-it notes and lifted a dog-eared copy of a *Cooking for Cancer* paperback from his chest where it had fallen, slowly, over the course of the night. And because it was cold outside as she pulled the front door gently closed behind her, pinching her bathrobe tight around her shoulders at the collarbone with her right hand and burying her left in one of its oversized pockets. Up the street, a neighbor's car sputtered and struggled to accelerate, turning onto the empty highway, heading north. She watched through the sharp crack of branches, grown almost leafless in the first real signs of winter. The morning, still gathering behind the long hills, thickened with trees. The air, still weighted with the unturned settling of frost. Her strength, a clean diffusion of gray light and undrawn breath, the silence— all distance in an unrhymed ache— a loneliness crafted from small filled hands and deeply loved days.

How much difference.

And I am lost in my

sameness.

The same birds, finches he thinks but doesn't know why,
          coming back each year to build nests between the glass
                    panels and the slightly frayed screen of their bedroom
                    window;

the tall fingers of their dogwood tapping the morning
          sky with wind, blown by winter storms; the last strands
                    of her hair, he would later find, tucked between dried
                    grass

and the plastic wrap from a cigarette pack,
          in a nest, lying beside their driveway – still chestnut, but brittle
                    as the bent brown spine last year's maple leaves in spring.

After the doctors, whose names he never did learn,
          had removed the first breast, her right, he felt desperate
                    to do something before she came home from the
                    hospital.

He carried everything he could out of the house to clean,
          scrubbed the floors, laundered the curtains,
                    patched old holes in the plaster walls.

Still, it wasn't enough. He thought about rescuing

    another dog, shopped for diamond pendants,

        searched the night sky for unnamed stars.

In the end, he painted their bedroom the color of lichen

    on a dead ash branch after rainfall, her favorite.

        The color, she had once pointed out

while they were walking in the park

    in May and had to take shelter from a sudden

        and momentary storm under a tree.

See, she had said, holding up a few flakes attached

    to a small, broken twig. *The way it's not quite green*

        but not all the way gray either. And it's not blue,

but kind of in between. I like it,

    she had whispered, her face close to his.

        It's not like anything else.

* * * * * *

Acknowledgements –

My thanks go out to *Naissance Press*, which published versions of many of this poem in a chapbook titled *Glory Glory*.

I would also like to thank my beautiful wife Ann for not only surviving these times with me but also teaching me more each day about what love means and deserves, Wanda Oakey of the Renascence House, members of the Illinois Poetry Society for giving me my first honest audience for these poems, Allison Smith for everything she did to help me understand the synthesis between creation and education, Bruce Beasley for what he taught me about the connection between grace and poetry, Frank Barthol for what he does to capture and display the beauty and dignity of forgotten people and places even when they are ugly. I would also like to thank an anonymous list of individuals who spent time talking about ideas that inspired these poems, or sat in silence with me in oncology waiting rooms at Vanderbilt Hospital in Nashville, Tennessee, Barnes Jewish Hospital in St. Louis, Missouri, and University of Chicago Hospital. You gave me the faith to believe someone wanted to hear what these poems have to say. Thank you as well to the nurses, custodial staff, food service workers, volunteers, physicians, pharmacists, and everyone else at these medical institutions who work diligently to make sure that patients and families can focus on the processes of healing and loss. Your work is often invisible but is not unappreciated.

Thank you, Sheridan.

Thank you, Mama.

Matthew Leavitt Brown is a writer, educator, and activist best known for his poetry and multimedia artwork that have been published and presented across North America and Europe. His work has been featured by a number of journals and presses and has been screened in film festivals, at universities, and at community forums. He holds degrees in writing from Southern Illinois University and Western Washington University as well as a PhD. in Composition, Rhetoric, and Language Studies from Middle Tennessee State University. His dissertation, scholarly research, and academic publishing deal with examining the neurocognitive-physiological-psychological ramifications of trauma along with common treatments. He uses this research to advocate for the use of expressive writing as a non-palliative treatment option for Post-tramatic Stress and its concurrent conditions.

He is the founder and facilitator of community literacy programs that help develop and advocate for the voices of individuals who have experienced trauma including veterans (*Writer Corps*), survivors of domestic and sexual violence (*The Lavinia Project*), and refugees and immigrants (*Nuestras Voces*). He currently teaches writing and literature at Middle Tennessee State University and lives with his wife, son, daughter, and beagle in Nashville.

Also by Matthew Brown:

Glory Glory (2012)
The River Sonnet (2014)

Visit the author's website at http://www.matthewbrownpoetry.com

Made in the USA
Lexington, KY
25 September 2018